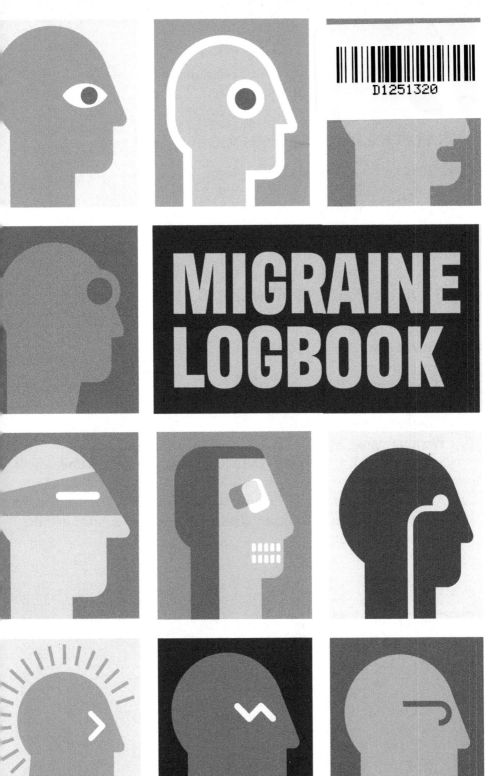

MIGRAINE LOGBOOK

MIGRAINE Tracker

Migraines are different for everyone. Record migraine attacks, symptoms and treatment to help prevent or minimize.

A migraine tracker can help:

- Help your doctor make a diagnosis
- Recognize triggers and warning signs
- Show migraine patterns
- Determine if medication is needed or if medication is working

Migraine tracker tracking includes:

- Date of migraine
- Time of day
- Day of the week
- Duration of migraine
- Severity of migraine
- Location of migraine
- Warning signs
- Symptoms such as dizziness, vertigo, sensitivity to light, sound, smells
- Medication
- Anything else that may be helpful. Such as side effects from medication, any potential triggers, stress, any changes in medication, and anything else that may be helpful

Step 1: Diary Overview

Step 2: Migraine Details

MIGRAINE LOGBOOK

DATE	NOTES	PAGE	INTENSITY				
			1	2	3	4	5
			☐	☐	☐	☐	☐
			☐	☐	☐	☐	☐
			☐	☐	☐	☐	☐
			☐	☐	☐	☐	☐
			☐	☐	☐	☐	☐
			☐	☐	☐	☐	☐
			☐	☐	☐	☐	☐
			☐	☐	☐	☐	☐
			☐	☐	☐	☐	☐
			☐	☐	☐	☐	☐
			☐	☐	☐	☐	☐
			☐	☐	☐	☐	☐
			☐	☐	☐	☐	☐
			☐	☐	☐	☐	☐
			☐	☐	☐	☐	☐
			☐	☐	☐	☐	☐
			☐	☐	☐	☐	☐
			☐	☐	☐	☐	☐
			☐	☐	☐	☐	☐
			☐	☐	☐	☐	☐
			☐	☐	☐	☐	☐
			☐	☐	☐	☐	☐
			☐	☐	☐	☐	☐
			☐	☐	☐	☐	☐
			☐	☐	☐	☐	☐
			☐	☐	☐	☐	☐

MIGRAINE LOGBOOK

DATE	NOTES	PAGE	INTENSITY
			1 2 3 4 5

INTENSITY
1 2 3 4 5

MIGRAINE LOGBOOK

DATE	NOTES	PAGE	INTENSITY				
			1	2	3	4	5
			☐	☐	☐	☐	☐
			☐	☐	☐	☐	☐
			☐	☐	☐	☐	☐
			☐	☐	☐	☐	☐
			☐	☐	☐	☐	☐
			☐	☐	☐	☐	☐
			☐	☐	☐	☐	☐
			☐	☐	☐	☐	☐
			☐	☐	☐	☐	☐
			☐	☐	☐	☐	☐
			☐	☐	☐	☐	☐
			☐	☐	☐	☐	☐
			☐	☐	☐	☐	☐
			☐	☐	☐	☐	☐
			☐	☐	☐	☐	☐
			☐	☐	☐	☐	☐
			☐	☐	☐	☐	☐
			☐	☐	☐	☐	☐
			☐	☐	☐	☐	☐
			☐	☐	☐	☐	☐
			☐	☐	☐	☐	☐
			☐	☐	☐	☐	☐
			☐	☐	☐	☐	☐
			☐	☐	☐	☐	☐
			☐	☐	☐	☐	☐
			☐	☐	☐	☐	☐

MIGRAINE LOGBOOK

DATE	NOTES	PAGE	INTENSITY
			1 2 3 4 5
			☐ ☐ ☐ ☐ ☐
			☐ ☐ ☐ ☐ ☐
			☐ ☐ ☐ ☐ ☐
			☐ ☐ ☐ ☐ ☐
			☐ ☐ ☐ ☐ ☐
			☐ ☐ ☐ ☐ ☐
			☐ ☐ ☐ ☐ ☐
			☐ ☐ ☐ ☐ ☐
			☐ ☐ ☐ ☐ ☐
			☐ ☐ ☐ ☐ ☐
			☐ ☐ ☐ ☐ ☐
			☐ ☐ ☐ ☐ ☐
			☐ ☐ ☐ ☐ ☐
			☐ ☐ ☐ ☐ ☐
			☐ ☐ ☐ ☐ ☐
			☐ ☐ ☐ ☐ ☐
			☐ ☐ ☐ ☐ ☐
			☐ ☐ ☐ ☐ ☐
			☐ ☐ ☐ ☐ ☐
			☐ ☐ ☐ ☐ ☐
			☐ ☐ ☐ ☐ ☐
			☐ ☐ ☐ ☐ ☐
			☐ ☐ ☐ ☐ ☐
			☐ ☐ ☐ ☐ ☐
			☐ ☐ ☐ ☐ ☐

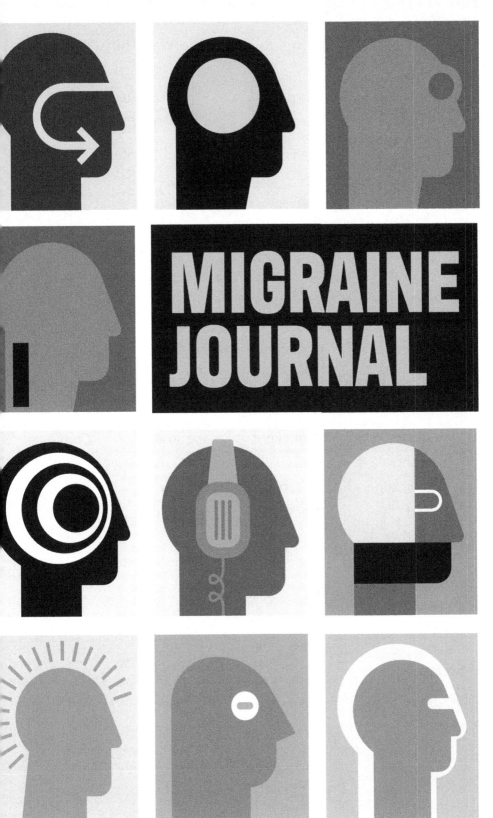

MIGRAINE JOURNAL

DATE	___ / ___ / ___	DAY	Mon	Tue	Wed	Thu	Fri	Sat	Sun

Time

Begin		End		Duration	
Begin		End		Duration	
Begin		End		Duration	

Location

☐ Tension ☐ Neck ☐ Migraine ☐ Cluster ☐ Sinus ☐ GCA

Severity

MILD ① ② ③ ④ ⑤ ⑥ ⑦ ⑧ ⑨ ⑩ SEVERE

Triggers

◯ Coffee	◯ Bright light	◯ Eye strain	◯ Commute
◯ Alcohol	◯ Stress	◯ Pc/Tv screen	◯ Pms
◯ Medication	◯ Anxiety	◯ Hunger	◯ Period
◯ Food	◯ Reading	◯ Insomnia	◯ Traveling
◯ Weather	◯ Noise	◯ Smell	◯
◯ Allergies	◯ Motion	◯ Sickness	◯

RELIEF MEASURES

Medication	
Water	
Sleep	
Exercise	
Other	

Notes

_____

_____

_____

8

Breakfast

_____
_____
_____
_____

Lunch

_____
_____
_____
_____

Dinner

_____
_____
_____
_____

Snacks/Drinks

_____
_____
_____
_____

Activities

Daily routine: Did you exercise, sleep, travel, etc.

_____
_____
_____
_____
_____
_____
_____
_____
_____
_____
_____

Notes

_____
_____
_____

DATE	___/___/___	DAY	Mon	Tue	Wed	Thu	Fri	Sat	Sun

Time

Begin		End		Duration	
Begin		End		Duration	
Begin		End		Duration	

Location

☐ Tension ☐ Neck ☐ Migraine ☐ Cluster ☐ Sinus ☐ GCA

Severity

MILD ① ② ③ ④ ⑤ ⑥ ⑦ ⑧ ⑨ ⑩ SEVERE

Triggers

◯ Coffee	◯ Bright light	◯ Eye strain	◯ Commute
◯ Alcohol	◯ Stress	◯ Pc/Tv screen	◯ Pms
◯ Medication	◯ Anxiety	◯ Hunger	◯ Period
◯ Food	◯ Reading	◯ Insomnia	◯ Traveling
◯ Weather	◯ Noise	◯ Smell	◯
◯ Allergies	◯ Motion	◯ Sickness	◯

RELIEF MEASURES

Medication	
Water	
Sleep	
Exercise	
Other	

Notes

_____
_____
_____

Breakfast

Lunch

Dinner

Snacks/Drinks

Daily routine: Did you exercise, sleep, travel, etc.

DATE ___/___/___	DAY	Mon	Tue	Wed	Thu	Fri	Sat	Sun

Time

Begin		End		Duration	
Begin		End		Duration	
Begin		End		Duration	

Location

☐ Tension ☐ Neck ☐ Migraine ☐ Cluster ☐ Sinus ☐ GCA

Severity

MILD ①②③④⑤⑥⑦⑧⑨⑩ SEVERE

Triggers

○ Coffee	○ Bright light	○ Eye strain	○ Commute
○ Alcohol	○ Stress	○ Pc/Tv screen	○ Pms
○ Medication	○ Anxiety	○ Hunger	○ Period
○ Food	○ Reading	○ Insomnia	○ Traveling
○ Weather	○ Noise	○ Smell	○
○ Allergies	○ Motion	○ Sickness	○

RELIEF MEASURES

Medication	
Water	
Sleep	
Exercise	
Other	

Notes

_____
_____
_____

Breakfast

_____
_____
_____
_____

Lunch

_____
_____
_____
_____

Dinner

_____
_____
_____
_____

Snacks/Drinks

_____
_____
_____
_____

Activities

Daily routine: Did you exercise, sleep, travel, etc.

_____
_____
_____
_____
_____
_____
_____
_____
_____
_____
_____

Notes

_____
_____
_____

DATE ___/___/___	DAY	Mon	Tue	Wed	Thu	Fri	Sat	Sun

Time

Begin		End		Duration	
Begin		End		Duration	
Begin		End		Duration	

Location

☐ Tension ☐ Neck ☐ Migraine ☐ Cluster ☐ Sinus ☐ GCA

Severity

MILD ① ② ③ ④ ⑤ ⑥ ⑦ ⑧ ⑨ ⑩ SEVERE

Triggers

○ Coffee	○ Bright light	○ Eye strain	○ Commute
○ Alcohol	○ Stress	○ Pc/Tv screen	○ Pms
○ Medication	○ Anxiety	○ Hunger	○ Period
○ Food	○ Reading	○ Insomnia	○ Traveling
○ Weather	○ Noise	○ Smell	○
○ Allergies	○ Motion	○ Sickness	○

RELIEF MEASURES

Medication	
Water	
Sleep	
Exercise	
Other	

Notes

_____
_____
_____
_____

Breakfast

_____
_____
_____
_____

Lunch

_____
_____
_____
_____

Dinner

_____
_____
_____
_____

Snacks/Drinks

_____
_____
_____
_____

Daily routine: Did you exercise, sleep, travel, etc.

_____
_____
_____
_____
_____
_____
_____
_____
_____
_____
_____
_____

_____
_____
_____

DATE ___/___/___	DAY	Mon	Tue	Wed	Thu	Fri	Sat	Sun

Time

Begin		End		Duration	
Begin		End		Duration	
Begin		End		Duration	

Location

☐ Tension ☐ Neck ☐ Migraine ☐ Cluster ☐ Sinus ☐ GCA

Severity

MILD ① ② ③ ④ ⑤ ⑥ ⑦ ⑧ ⑨ ⑩ SEVERE

Triggers

○ Coffee	○ Bright light	○ Eye strain	○ Commute
○ Alcohol	○ Stress	○ Pc/Tv screen	○ Pms
○ Medication	○ Anxiety	○ Hunger	○ Period
○ Food	○ Reading	○ Insomnia	○ Traveling
○ Weather	○ Noise	○ Smell	○
○ Allergies	○ Motion	○ Sickness	○

RELIEF MEASURES

Medication	
Water	
Sleep	
Exercise	
Other	

Notes

_____
_____
_____
_____

Breakfast

Lunch

Dinner

Snacks/Drinks

Daily routine: Did you exercise, sleep, travel, etc.

DATE ___/___/___	DAY	Mon	Tue	Wed	Thu	Fri	Sat	Sun

Time

Begin		End		Duration	
Begin		End		Duration	
Begin		End		Duration	

Location

☐ Tension   ☐ Neck   ☐ Migraine   ☐ Cluster   ☐ Sinus   ☐ GCA

Severity

MILD ①②③④⑤⑥⑦⑧⑨⑩ SEVERE

Triggers

○ Coffee	○ Bright light	○ Eye strain	○ Commute
○ Alcohol	○ Stress	○ Pc/Tv screen	○ Pms
○ Medication	○ Anxiety	○ Hunger	○ Period
○ Food	○ Reading	○ Insomnia	○ Traveling
○ Weather	○ Noise	○ Smell	○
○ Allergies	○ Motion	○ Sickness	○

RELIEF MEASURES

Medication	
Water	
Sleep	
Exercise	
Other	

Notes

_____
_____
_____
_____

Breakfast

_____
_____
_____
_____

Lunch

_____
_____
_____
_____

Dinner

_____
_____
_____
_____

Snacks/Drinks

_____
_____
_____
_____

Activities

Daily routine: Did you exercise, sleep, travel, etc.

_____
_____
_____
_____
_____
_____
_____
_____
_____
_____
_____

Notes

_____
_____
_____

DATE	___/___/___	DAY	Mon	Tue	Wed	Thu	Fri	Sat	Sun

Time

Begin		End		Duration	
Begin		End		Duration	
Begin		End		Duration	

Location

☐ Tension ☐ Neck ☐ Migraine ☐ Cluster ☐ Sinus ☐ GCA

Severity

MILD ① ② ③ ④ ⑤ ⑥ ⑦ ⑧ ⑨ ⑩ SEVERE

Triggers

○ Coffee	○ Bright light	○ Eye strain	○ Commute
○ Alcohol	○ Stress	○ Pc/Tv screen	○ Pms
○ Medication	○ Anxiety	○ Hunger	○ Period
○ Food	○ Reading	○ Insomnia	○ Traveling
○ Weather	○ Noise	○ Smell	○
○ Allergies	○ Motion	○ Sickness	○

RELIEF MEASURES

Medication	
Water	
Sleep	
Exercise	
Other	

Notes

_____
_____
_____

Breakfast

_____
_____
_____
_____

Lunch

_____
_____
_____
_____

Dinner

_____
_____
_____
_____

Snacks/Drinks

_____
_____
_____
_____

Activities

Daily routine: Did you exercise, sleep, travel, etc.

_____
_____
_____
_____
_____
_____
_____
_____
_____
_____
_____

Notes

_____
_____
_____

DATE ___/___/___	DAY	Mon	Tue	Wed	Thu	Fri	Sat	Sun

Time

Begin		End		Duration	
Begin		End		Duration	
Begin		End		Duration	

Location

☐ Tension ☐ Neck ☐ Migraine ☐ Cluster ☐ Sinus ☐ GCA

Severity

MILD ① ② ③ ④ ⑤ ⑥ ⑦ ⑧ ⑨ ⑩ SEVERE

Triggers

○ Coffee	○ Bright light	○ Eye strain	○ Commute
○ Alcohol	○ Stress	○ Pc/Tv screen	○ Pms
○ Medication	○ Anxiety	○ Hunger	○ Period
○ Food	○ Reading	○ Insomnia	○ Traveling
○ Weather	○ Noise	○ Smell	○
○ Allergies	○ Motion	○ Sickness	○

RELIEF MEASURES

Medication	
Water	
Sleep	
Exercise	
Other	

Notes

_____
_____
_____
_____

Breakfast

_____
_____
_____

Lunch

_____
_____
_____

Dinner

_____
_____
_____

Snacks/Drinks

_____
_____
_____

Activities

Daily routine: Did you exercise, sleep, travel, etc.

_____
_____
_____
_____
_____
_____
_____
_____
_____

Notes

_____
_____
_____

DATE	/ /	DAY	Mon	Tue	Wed	Thu	Fri	Sat	Sun

Time

Begin		End		Duration	
Begin		End		Duration	
Begin		End		Duration	

Location

☐ Tension ☐ Neck ☐ Migraine ☐ Cluster ☐ Sinus ☐ GCA

Severity

MILD (1) (2) (3) (4) (5) (6) (7) (8) (9) (10) SEVERE

Triggers

○ Coffee	○ Bright light	○ Eye strain	○ Commute
○ Alcohol	○ Stress	○ Pc/Tv screen	○ Pms
○ Medication	○ Anxiety	○ Hunger	○ Period
○ Food	○ Reading	○ Insomnia	○ Traveling
○ Weather	○ Noise	○ Smell	○
○ Allergies	○ Motion	○ Sickness	○

RELIEF MEASURES

Medication	
Water	
Sleep	
Exercise	
Other	

Notes

_____
_____
_____

24

Breakfast

_____
_____
_____
_____

Lunch

_____
_____
_____
_____

Dinner

_____
_____
_____
_____

Snacks/Drinks

_____
_____
_____
_____

Activities

Daily routine: Did you exercise, sleep, travel, etc.

_____
_____
_____
_____
_____
_____
_____
_____
_____
_____
_____
_____

Notes

_____
_____
_____

| DATE ___ / ___ / ___ | DAY | Mon | Tue | Wed | Thu | Fri | Sat | Sun |

Time

Begin		End		Duration	
Begin		End		Duration	
Begin		End		Duration	

Location

☐ Tension ☐ Neck ☐ Migraine ☐ Cluster ☐ Sinus ☐ GCA

Severity

MILD ① ② ③ ④ ⑤ ⑥ ⑦ ⑧ ⑨ ⑩ SEVERE

Triggers

○ Coffee	○ Bright light	○ Eye strain	○ Commute
○ Alcohol	○ Stress	○ Pc/Tv screen	○ Pms
○ Medication	○ Anxiety	○ Hunger	○ Period
○ Food	○ Reading	○ Insomnia	○ Traveling
○ Weather	○ Noise	○ Smell	○
○ Allergies	○ Motion	○ Sickness	○

RELIEF MEASURES

Medication	
Water	
Sleep	
Exercise	
Other	

Notes

_____
_____
_____

Breakfast

Lunch

Dinner

Snacks/Drinks

Daily routine: Did you exercise, sleep, travel, etc.

DATE ___ / ___ / ___	DAY	Mon	Tue	Wed	Thu	Fri	Sat	Sun

Time

Begin		End		Duration	
Begin		End		Duration	
Begin		End		Duration	

Location

☐ Tension ☐ Neck ☐ Migraine ☐ Cluster ☐ Sinus ☐ GCA

Severity

MILD ① ② ③ ④ ⑤ ⑥ ⑦ ⑧ ⑨ ⑩ SEVERE

Triggers

○ Coffee	○ Bright light	○ Eye strain	○ Commute
○ Alcohol	○ Stress	○ Pc/Tv screen	○ Pms
○ Medication	○ Anxiety	○ Hunger	○ Period
○ Food	○ Reading	○ Insomnia	○ Traveling
○ Weather	○ Noise	○ Smell	○
○ Allergies	○ Motion	○ Sickness	○

RELIEF MEASURES

Medication	
Water	
Sleep	
Exercise	
Other	

Notes

_____
_____
_____
_____

Breakfast

_____
_____
_____
_____

Lunch

_____
_____
_____
_____

Dinner

_____
_____
_____
_____

Snacks/Drinks

_____
_____
_____
_____

Activities

Daily routine: Did you exercise, sleep, travel, etc.

_____
_____
_____
_____
_____
_____
_____
_____
_____
_____
_____

Notes

_____
_____
_____

Time

Begin		End		Duration	
Begin		End		Duration	
Begin		End		Duration	

Location

☐ Tension   ☐ Neck   ☐ Migraine   ☐ Cluster   ☐ Sinus   ☐ GCA

Severity

MILD ① ② ③ ④ ⑤ ⑥ ⑦ ⑧ ⑨ ⑩ SEVERE

Triggers

○ Coffee	○ Bright light	○ Eye strain	○ Commute
○ Alcohol	○ Stress	○ Pc/Tv screen	○ Pms
○ Medication	○ Anxiety	○ Hunger	○ Period
○ Food	○ Reading	○ Insomnia	○ Traveling
○ Weather	○ Noise	○ Smell	○
○ Allergies	○ Motion	○ Sickness	○

RELIEF MEASURES

Medication	
Water	
Sleep	
Exercise	
Other	

Notes

_____
_____
_____

Breakfast

_____
_____
_____
_____

Lunch

_____
_____
_____
_____

Dinner

_____
_____
_____
_____

Snacks/Drinks

_____
_____
_____
_____

Activities

Daily routine: Did you exercise, sleep, travel, etc.

_____
_____
_____
_____
_____
_____
_____
_____
_____
_____
_____

Notes

_____
_____
_____

DATE ___/___/___	DAY	Mon	Tue	Wed	Thu	Fri	Sat	Sun

Time

Begin		End		Duration	
Begin		End		Duration	
Begin		End		Duration	

Location

☐ Tension ☐ Neck ☐ Migraine ☐ Cluster ☐ Sinus ☐ GCA

Severity

MILD ① ② ③ ④ ⑤ ⑥ ⑦ ⑧ ⑨ ⑩ SEVERE

Triggers

○ Coffee	○ Bright light	○ Eye strain	○ Commute
○ Alcohol	○ Stress	○ Pc/Tv screen	○ Pms
○ Medication	○ Anxiety	○ Hunger	○ Period
○ Food	○ Reading	○ Insomnia	○ Traveling
○ Weather	○ Noise	○ Smell	○
○ Allergies	○ Motion	○ Sickness	○

RELIEF MEASURES

Medication	
Water	
Sleep	
Exercise	
Other	

Notes

_____
_____
_____
_____

32

Breakfast

_____
_____
_____
_____

Lunch

_____
_____
_____
_____

Dinner

_____
_____
_____
_____

Snacks/Drinks

_____
_____
_____
_____

Activities

Daily routine: Did you exercise, sleep, travel, etc.

_____
_____
_____
_____
_____
_____
_____
_____
_____
_____
_____

Notes

_____
_____
_____

| DATE ___/___/___ | DAY | Mon | Tue | Wed | Thu | Fri | Sat | Sun |

Time

Begin		End		Duration	
Begin		End		Duration	
Begin		End		Duration	

Location

☐ Tension ☐ Neck ☐ Migraine ☐ Cluster ☐ Sinus ☐ GCA

Severity

MILD ①②③④⑤⑥⑦⑧⑨⑩ SEVERE

Triggers

○ Coffee	○ Bright light	○ Eye strain	○ Commute
○ Alcohol	○ Stress	○ Pc/Tv screen	○ Pms
○ Medication	○ Anxiety	○ Hunger	○ Period
○ Food	○ Reading	○ Insomnia	○ Traveling
○ Weather	○ Noise	○ Smell	○
○ Allergies	○ Motion	○ Sickness	○

RELIEF MEASURES

Medication	
Water	
Sleep	
Exercise	
Other	

Notes

_____
_____
_____
_____

34

Breakfast

_____
_____
_____
_____

Lunch

_____
_____
_____
_____

Dinner

_____
_____
_____
_____

Snacks/Drinks

_____
_____
_____
_____

Activities

Daily routine: Did you exercise, sleep, travel, etc.

_____
_____
_____
_____
_____
_____
_____
_____
_____
_____
_____

Notes

_____
_____
_____

DATE	___/___/___	DAY	Mon	Tue	Wed	Thu	Fri	Sat	Sun

Time

Begin		End		Duration	
Begin		End		Duration	
Begin		End		Duration	

Location

- ☐ Tension
- ☐ Neck
- ☐ Migraine
- ☐ Cluster
- ☐ Sinus
- ☐ GCA

Severity

MILD ① ② ③ ④ ⑤ ⑥ ⑦ ⑧ ⑨ ⑩ SEVERE

Triggers

◯ Coffee	◯ Bright light	◯ Eye strain	◯ Commute
◯ Alcohol	◯ Stress	◯ Pc/Tv screen	◯ Pms
◯ Medication	◯ Anxiety	◯ Hunger	◯ Period
◯ Food	◯ Reading	◯ Insomnia	◯ Traveling
◯ Weather	◯ Noise	◯ Smell	◯
◯ Allergies	◯ Motion	◯ Sickness	◯

RELIEF MEASURES

Medication	
Water	
Sleep	
Exercise	
Other	

Notes

_____
_____
_____

Breakfast

Lunch

Dinner

Snacks/Drinks

Daily routine: Did you exercise, sleep, travel, etc.

DATE ___/___/___	DAY	Mon	Tue	Wed	Thu	Fri	Sat	Sun

Time

Begin		End		Duration	
Begin		End		Duration	
Begin		End		Duration	

Location

☐ Tension ☐ Neck ☐ Migraine ☐ Cluster ☐ Sinus ☐ GCA

Severity

MILD ① ② ③ ④ ⑤ ⑥ ⑦ ⑧ ⑨ ⑩ SEVERE

Triggers

○ Coffee	○ Bright light	○ Eye strain	○ Commute
○ Alcohol	○ Stress	○ Pc/Tv screen	○ Pms
○ Medication	○ Anxiety	○ Hunger	○ Period
○ Food	○ Reading	○ Insomnia	○ Traveling
○ Weather	○ Noise	○ Smell	○
○ Allergies	○ Motion	○ Sickness	○

RELIEF MEASURES

Medication	
Water	
Sleep	
Exercise	
Other	

Notes

Eating Log

Breakfast

Lunch

Dinner

Snacks/Drinks

Activities

Daily routine: Did you exercise, sleep, travel, etc.

Notes

DATE	___/___/___	DAY	Mon	Tue	Wed	Thu	Fri	Sat	Sun

Time

Begin		End		Duration	
Begin		End		Duration	
Begin		End		Duration	

Location

☐ Tension ☐ Neck ☐ Migraine ☐ Cluster ☐ Sinus ☐ GCA

Severity

MILD ① ② ③ ④ ⑤ ⑥ ⑦ ⑧ ⑨ ⑩ SEVERE

Triggers

◯ Coffee	◯ Bright light	◯ Eye strain	◯ Commute
◯ Alcohol	◯ Stress	◯ Pc/Tv screen	◯ Pms
◯ Medication	◯ Anxiety	◯ Hunger	◯ Period
◯ Food	◯ Reading	◯ Insomnia	◯ Traveling
◯ Weather	◯ Noise	◯ Smell	◯
◯ Allergies	◯ Motion	◯ Sickness	◯

RELIEF MEASURES

Medication	
Water	
Sleep	
Exercise	
Other	

Notes

_____
_____
_____
_____

40

Breakfast

_____

_____

_____

_____

Lunch

_____

_____

_____

_____

Dinner

_____

_____

_____

_____

Snacks/Drinks

_____

_____

_____

_____

Activities

Daily routine: Did you exercise, sleep, travel, etc.

_____

_____

_____

_____

_____

_____

_____

_____

_____

_____

_____

Notes

_____

_____

_____

DATE	/ /	DAY	Mon	Tue	Wed	Thu	Fri	Sat	Sun

Time

Begin		End		Duration	
Begin		End		Duration	
Begin		End		Duration	

Location

☐ Tension ☐ Neck ☐ Migraine ☐ Cluster ☐ Sinus ☐ GCA

Severity

MILD ① ② ③ ④ ⑤ ⑥ ⑦ ⑧ ⑨ ⑩ SEVERE

Triggers

◯ Coffee	◯ Bright light	◯ Eye strain	◯ Commute
◯ Alcohol	◯ Stress	◯ Pc/Tv screen	◯ Pms
◯ Medication	◯ Anxiety	◯ Hunger	◯ Period
◯ Food	◯ Reading	◯ Insomnia	◯ Traveling
◯ Weather	◯ Noise	◯ Smell	◯
◯ Allergies	◯ Motion	◯ Sickness	◯

RELIEF MEASURES

Medication	
Water	
Sleep	
Exercise	
Other	

Notes

_____
_____
_____

Breakfast

_____
_____
_____
_____

Lunch

_____
_____
_____
_____

Dinner

_____
_____
_____
_____

Snacks/Drinks

_____
_____
_____
_____

Daily routine: Did you exercise, sleep, travel, etc.

_____
_____
_____
_____
_____
_____
_____
_____
_____
_____
_____
_____

_____
_____
_____

DATE	___ / ___ / ___	DAY	Mon	Tue	Wed	Thu	Fri	Sat	Sun

Time

Begin		End		Duration	
Begin		End		Duration	
Begin		End		Duration	

Location

☐ Tension ☐ Neck ☐ Migraine ☐ Cluster ☐ Sinus ☐ GCA

Severity

MILD ① ② ③ ④ ⑤ ⑥ ⑦ ⑧ ⑨ ⑩ SEVERE

Triggers

○ Coffee	○ Bright light	○ Eye strain	○ Commute
○ Alcohol	○ Stress	○ Pc/Tv screen	○ Pms
○ Medication	○ Anxiety	○ Hunger	○ Period
○ Food	○ Reading	○ Insomnia	○ Traveling
○ Weather	○ Noise	○ Smell	○
○ Allergies	○ Motion	○ Sickness	○

RELIEF MEASURES

Medication	
Water	
Sleep	
Exercise	
Other	

Notes

_____
_____
_____

Breakfast

_____
_____
_____

Lunch

_____
_____
_____

Dinner

_____
_____
_____

Snacks/Drinks

_____
_____
_____
_____

Activities

Daily routine: Did you exercise, sleep, travel, etc.

_____
_____
_____
_____
_____
_____
_____
_____
_____
_____
_____

Notes

_____
_____
_____

DATE	___ / ___ / ___	DAY	Mon	Tue	Wed	Thu	Fri	Sat	Sun

Time

Begin		End		Duration	
Begin		End		Duration	
Begin		End		Duration	

Location

☐ Tension ☐ Neck ☐ Migraine ☐ Cluster ☐ Sinus ☐ GCA

Severity

MILD ① ② ③ ④ ⑤ ⑥ ⑦ ⑧ ⑨ ⑩ SEVERE

Triggers

○ Coffee	○ Bright light	○ Eye strain	○ Commute
○ Alcohol	○ Stress	○ Pc/Tv screen	○ Pms
○ Medication	○ Anxiety	○ Hunger	○ Period
○ Food	○ Reading	○ Insomnia	○ Traveling
○ Weather	○ Noise	○ Smell	○
○ Allergies	○ Motion	○ Sickness	○

RELIEF MEASURES

Medication	
Water	
Sleep	
Exercise	
Other	

Notes

_____
_____
_____
_____

Breakfast

Lunch

Dinner

Snacks/Drinks

Daily routine: Did you exercise, sleep, travel, etc.

DATE ___ / ___ / ___	DAY	Mon	Tue	Wed	Thu	Fri	Sat	Sun

Time

Begin		End		Duration	
Begin		End		Duration	
Begin		End		Duration	

Location

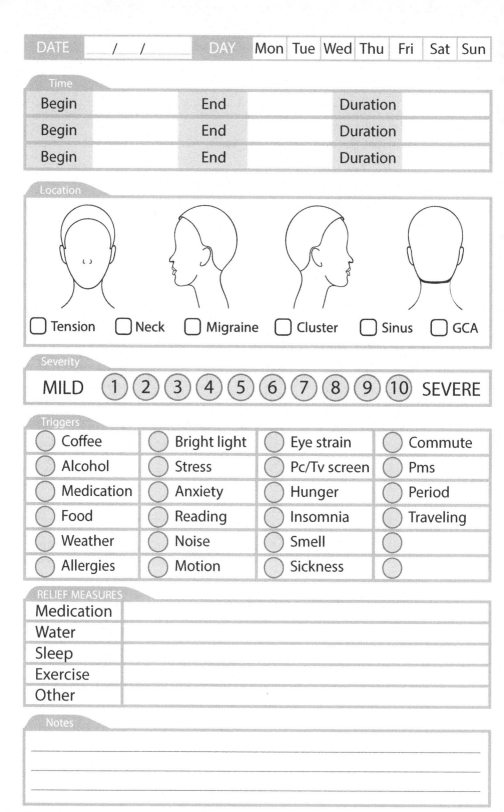

☐ Tension ☐ Neck ☐ Migraine ☐ Cluster ☐ Sinus ☐ GCA

Severity

MILD ① ② ③ ④ ⑤ ⑥ ⑦ ⑧ ⑨ ⑩ SEVERE

Triggers

◯ Coffee	◯ Bright light	◯ Eye strain	◯ Commute
◯ Alcohol	◯ Stress	◯ Pc/Tv screen	◯ Pms
◯ Medication	◯ Anxiety	◯ Hunger	◯ Period
◯ Food	◯ Reading	◯ Insomnia	◯ Traveling
◯ Weather	◯ Noise	◯ Smell	◯
◯ Allergies	◯ Motion	◯ Sickness	◯

RELIEF MEASURES

Medication	
Water	
Sleep	
Exercise	
Other	

Notes

_____
_____
_____

Breakfast

Lunch

Dinner

Snacks/Drinks

Daily routine: Did you exercise, sleep, travel, etc.

DATE ___/___/___	DAY	Mon	Tue	Wed	Thu	Fri	Sat	Sun

Time

Begin		End		Duration	
Begin		End		Duration	
Begin		End		Duration	

Location

☐ Tension ☐ Neck ☐ Migraine ☐ Cluster ☐ Sinus ☐ GCA

Severity

MILD ① ② ③ ④ ⑤ ⑥ ⑦ ⑧ ⑨ ⑩ SEVERE

Triggers

○ Coffee	○ Bright light	○ Eye strain	○ Commute
○ Alcohol	○ Stress	○ Pc/Tv screen	○ Pms
○ Medication	○ Anxiety	○ Hunger	○ Period
○ Food	○ Reading	○ Insomnia	○ Traveling
○ Weather	○ Noise	○ Smell	○
○ Allergies	○ Motion	○ Sickness	○

RELIEF MEASURES

Medication	
Water	
Sleep	
Exercise	
Other	

Notes

_____
_____
_____

50

Breakfast

_____
_____
_____
_____

Lunch

_____
_____
_____
_____

Dinner

_____
_____
_____
_____

Snacks/Drinks

_____
_____
_____
_____
_____

Activities

Daily routine: Did you exercise, sleep, travel, etc.

_____
_____
_____
_____
_____
_____
_____
_____
_____
_____
_____
_____
_____

Notes

_____
_____
_____

DATE ___/___/___	DAY	Mon	Tue	Wed	Thu	Fri	Sat	Sun

Time

Begin		End		Duration	
Begin		End		Duration	
Begin		End		Duration	

Location

☐ Tension ☐ Neck ☐ Migraine ☐ Cluster ☐ Sinus ☐ GCA

Severity

MILD ① ② ③ ④ ⑤ ⑥ ⑦ ⑧ ⑨ ⑩ SEVERE

Triggers

○ Coffee	○ Bright light	○ Eye strain	○ Commute
○ Alcohol	○ Stress	○ Pc/Tv screen	○ Pms
○ Medication	○ Anxiety	○ Hunger	○ Period
○ Food	○ Reading	○ Insomnia	○ Traveling
○ Weather	○ Noise	○ Smell	○
○ Allergies	○ Motion	○ Sickness	○

RELIEF MEASURES

Medication	
Water	
Sleep	
Exercise	
Other	

Notes

_____
_____
_____

Breakfast

_____
_____
_____
_____

Lunch

_____
_____
_____
_____

Dinner

_____
_____
_____
_____

Snacks/Drinks

_____
_____
_____
_____

Activities

Daily routine: Did you exercise, sleep, travel, etc.

_____
_____
_____
_____
_____
_____
_____
_____
_____
_____

Notes

_____
_____
_____

DATE	/ /	DAY	Mon	Tue	Wed	Thu	Fri	Sat	Sun

Time

Begin		End		Duration	
Begin		End		Duration	
Begin		End		Duration	

Location

☐ Tension ☐ Neck ☐ Migraine ☐ Cluster ☐ Sinus ☐ GCA

Severity

MILD ① ② ③ ④ ⑤ ⑥ ⑦ ⑧ ⑨ ⑩ SEVERE

Triggers

○ Coffee	○ Bright light	○ Eye strain	○ Commute
○ Alcohol	○ Stress	○ Pc/Tv screen	○ Pms
○ Medication	○ Anxiety	○ Hunger	○ Period
○ Food	○ Reading	○ Insomnia	○ Traveling
○ Weather	○ Noise	○ Smell	○
○ Allergies	○ Motion	○ Sickness	○

RELIEF MEASURES

Medication	
Water	
Sleep	
Exercise	
Other	

Notes

_____
_____
_____
_____

Breakfast

_____
_____
_____
_____

Lunch

_____
_____
_____

Dinner

_____
_____
_____

Snacks/Drinks

_____
_____
_____
_____

Daily routine: Did you exercise, sleep, travel, etc.

_____
_____
_____
_____
_____
_____
_____
_____
_____
_____
_____
_____
_____

_____
_____
_____

DATE	___ / ___ / ___	DAY	Mon	Tue	Wed	Thu	Fri	Sat	Sun

Time

Begin		End		Duration	
Begin		End		Duration	
Begin		End		Duration	

Location

☐ Tension ☐ Neck ☐ Migraine ☐ Cluster ☐ Sinus ☐ GCA

Severity

MILD ① ② ③ ④ ⑤ ⑥ ⑦ ⑧ ⑨ ⑩ SEVERE

Triggers

○ Coffee	○ Bright light	○ Eye strain	○ Commute
○ Alcohol	○ Stress	○ Pc/Tv screen	○ Pms
○ Medication	○ Anxiety	○ Hunger	○ Period
○ Food	○ Reading	○ Insomnia	○ Traveling
○ Weather	○ Noise	○ Smell	○
○ Allergies	○ Motion	○ Sickness	○

RELIEF MEASURES

Medication	
Water	
Sleep	
Exercise	
Other	

Notes

_____
_____
_____
_____

Breakfast

_____
_____
_____
_____

Lunch

_____
_____
_____
_____

Dinner

_____
_____
_____
_____

Snacks/Drinks

_____
_____
_____
_____

Activities

Daily routine: Did you exercise, sleep, travel, etc.

_____
_____
_____
_____
_____
_____
_____
_____
_____
_____
_____

Notes

_____
_____
_____

| DATE | ___ / ___ / ___ | DAY | Mon | Tue | Wed | Thu | Fri | Sat | Sun |

Time

Begin		End		Duration	
Begin		End		Duration	
Begin		End		Duration	

Location

☐ Tension ☐ Neck ☐ Migraine ☐ Cluster ☐ Sinus ☐ GCA

Severity

MILD ① ② ③ ④ ⑤ ⑥ ⑦ ⑧ ⑨ ⑩ SEVERE

Triggers

○ Coffee	○ Bright light	○ Eye strain	○ Commute
○ Alcohol	○ Stress	○ Pc/Tv screen	○ Pms
○ Medication	○ Anxiety	○ Hunger	○ Period
○ Food	○ Reading	○ Insomnia	○ Traveling
○ Weather	○ Noise	○ Smell	○
○ Allergies	○ Motion	○ Sickness	○

RELIEF MEASURES

Medication	
Water	
Sleep	
Exercise	
Other	

Notes

_____

_____

_____

Breakfast

_____
_____
_____
_____

Lunch

_____
_____
_____
_____

Dinner

_____
_____
_____
_____

Snacks/Drinks

_____
_____
_____
_____

Activities

Daily routine: Did you exercise, sleep, travel, etc.

_____
_____
_____
_____
_____
_____
_____
_____
_____
_____
_____

Notes

_____
_____
_____

DATE ___/___/___	DAY	Mon	Tue	Wed	Thu	Fri	Sat	Sun

Time

Begin		End		Duration	
Begin		End		Duration	
Begin		End		Duration	

Location

☐ Tension ☐ Neck ☐ Migraine ☐ Cluster ☐ Sinus ☐ GCA

Severity

MILD ①②③④⑤⑥⑦⑧⑨⑩ SEVERE

Triggers

○ Coffee	○ Bright light	○ Eye strain	○ Commute
○ Alcohol	○ Stress	○ Pc/Tv screen	○ Pms
○ Medication	○ Anxiety	○ Hunger	○ Period
○ Food	○ Reading	○ Insomnia	○ Traveling
○ Weather	○ Noise	○ Smell	○
○ Allergies	○ Motion	○ Sickness	○

RELIEF MEASURES

Medication	
Water	
Sleep	
Exercise	
Other	

Notes

_____
_____
_____

Breakfast

_____
_____
_____
_____

Lunch

_____
_____
_____
_____

Dinner

_____
_____
_____
_____

Snacks/Drinks

_____
_____
_____
_____

Activities

Daily routine: Did you exercise, sleep, travel, etc.

_____
_____
_____
_____
_____
_____
_____
_____
_____
_____
_____

Notes

_____
_____
_____
_____

DATE ___ / ___ / ___	DAY	Mon	Tue	Wed	Thu	Fri	Sat	Sun

Time

Begin		End		Duration	
Begin		End		Duration	
Begin		End		Duration	

Location

☐ Tension ☐ Neck ☐ Migraine ☐ Cluster ☐ Sinus ☐ GCA

Severity

MILD (1) (2) (3) (4) (5) (6) (7) (8) (9) (10) SEVERE

Triggers

○ Coffee	○ Bright light	○ Eye strain	○ Commute
○ Alcohol	○ Stress	○ Pc/Tv screen	○ Pms
○ Medication	○ Anxiety	○ Hunger	○ Period
○ Food	○ Reading	○ Insomnia	○ Traveling
○ Weather	○ Noise	○ Smell	○
○ Allergies	○ Motion	○ Sickness	○

RELIEF MEASURES

Medication	
Water	
Sleep	
Exercise	
Other	

Notes

_____
_____
_____
_____

Breakfast

_____
_____
_____
_____

Lunch

_____
_____
_____
_____

Dinner

_____
_____
_____
_____

Snacks/Drinks

_____
_____
_____
_____

Activities

Daily routine: Did you exercise, sleep, travel, etc.

_____
_____
_____
_____
_____
_____
_____
_____
_____
_____
_____

Notes

_____
_____
_____

DATE	___ / ___ / ___	DAY	Mon	Tue	Wed	Thu	Fri	Sat	Sun

Time

Begin		End		Duration	
Begin		End		Duration	
Begin		End		Duration	

Location

☐ Tension ☐ Neck ☐ Migraine ☐ Cluster ☐ Sinus ☐ GCA

Severity

MILD ① ② ③ ④ ⑤ ⑥ ⑦ ⑧ ⑨ ⑩ SEVERE

Triggers

◯ Coffee	◯ Bright light	◯ Eye strain	◯ Commute
◯ Alcohol	◯ Stress	◯ Pc/Tv screen	◯ Pms
◯ Medication	◯ Anxiety	◯ Hunger	◯ Period
◯ Food	◯ Reading	◯ Insomnia	◯ Traveling
◯ Weather	◯ Noise	◯ Smell	◯
◯ Allergies	◯ Motion	◯ Sickness	◯

RELIEF MEASURES

Medication	
Water	
Sleep	
Exercise	
Other	

Notes

Breakfast

_____
_____
_____
_____

Lunch

_____
_____
_____
_____

Dinner

_____
_____
_____
_____

Snacks/Drinks

_____
_____
_____
_____

Activities

Daily routine: Did you exercise, sleep, travel, etc.

_____
_____
_____
_____
_____
_____
_____
_____
_____
_____

Notes

_____
_____
_____

DATE	___/___/___	DAY	Mon	Tue	Wed	Thu	Fri	Sat	Sun

Time

Begin		End		Duration	
Begin		End		Duration	
Begin		End		Duration	

Location

☐ Tension ☐ Neck ☐ Migraine ☐ Cluster ☐ Sinus ☐ GCA

Severity

MILD ① ② ③ ④ ⑤ ⑥ ⑦ ⑧ ⑨ ⑩ SEVERE

Triggers

◯ Coffee	◯ Bright light	◯ Eye strain	◯ Commute
◯ Alcohol	◯ Stress	◯ Pc/Tv screen	◯ Pms
◯ Medication	◯ Anxiety	◯ Hunger	◯ Period
◯ Food	◯ Reading	◯ Insomnia	◯ Traveling
◯ Weather	◯ Noise	◯ Smell	◯
◯ Allergies	◯ Motion	◯ Sickness	◯

RELIEF MEASURES

Medication	
Water	
Sleep	
Exercise	
Other	

Notes

_____

_____

_____

Breakfast

_____
_____
_____
_____

Lunch

_____
_____
_____
_____

Dinner

_____
_____
_____
_____

Snacks/Drinks

_____
_____
_____
_____

Activities

Daily routine: Did you exercise, sleep, travel, etc.

_____
_____
_____
_____
_____
_____
_____
_____
_____
_____
_____

Notes

_____
_____
_____

DATE ___ / ___ / ___	DAY	Mon	Tue	Wed	Thu	Fri	Sat	Sun

Time

Begin		End		Duration	
Begin		End		Duration	
Begin		End		Duration	

Location

☐ Tension ☐ Neck ☐ Migraine ☐ Cluster ☐ Sinus ☐ GCA

Severity

MILD (1) (2) (3) (4) (5) (6) (7) (8) (9) (10) SEVERE

Triggers

○ Coffee	○ Bright light	○ Eye strain	○ Commute
○ Alcohol	○ Stress	○ Pc/Tv screen	○ Pms
○ Medication	○ Anxiety	○ Hunger	○ Period
○ Food	○ Reading	○ Insomnia	○ Traveling
○ Weather	○ Noise	○ Smell	○
○ Allergies	○ Motion	○ Sickness	○

RELIEF MEASURES

Medication	
Water	
Sleep	
Exercise	
Other	

Notes

_____
_____
_____
_____

Breakfast

Lunch

Dinner

Snacks/Drinks

Daily routine: Did you exercise, sleep, travel, etc.

DATE ___/___/___	DAY	Mon	Tue	Wed	Thu	Fri	Sat	Sun

Time

Begin		End		Duration	
Begin		End		Duration	
Begin		End		Duration	

Location

☐ Tension ☐ Neck ☐ Migraine ☐ Cluster ☐ Sinus ☐ GCA

Severity

MILD ①②③④⑤⑥⑦⑧⑨⑩ SEVERE

Triggers

○ Coffee	○ Bright light	○ Eye strain	○ Commute
○ Alcohol	○ Stress	○ Pc/Tv screen	○ Pms
○ Medication	○ Anxiety	○ Hunger	○ Period
○ Food	○ Reading	○ Insomnia	○ Traveling
○ Weather	○ Noise	○ Smell	○
○ Allergies	○ Motion	○ Sickness	○

RELIEF MEASURES

Medication	
Water	
Sleep	
Exercise	
Other	

Notes

_____
_____
_____

Breakfast

_____
_____
_____
_____

Lunch

_____
_____
_____
_____

Dinner

_____
_____
_____

Snacks/Drinks

_____
_____
_____
_____

Activities

Daily routine: Did you exercise, sleep, travel, etc.

_____
_____
_____
_____
_____
_____
_____
_____
_____
_____

Notes

_____
_____
_____

DATE	___/___/___	DAY	Mon	Tue	Wed	Thu	Fri	Sat	Sun

Time

Begin		End		Duration	
Begin		End		Duration	
Begin		End		Duration	

Location

☐ Tension ☐ Neck ☐ Migraine ☐ Cluster ☐ Sinus ☐ GCA

Severity

MILD ①②③④⑤⑥⑦⑧⑨⑩ SEVERE

Triggers

○ Coffee	○ Bright light	○ Eye strain	○ Commute
○ Alcohol	○ Stress	○ Pc/Tv screen	○ Pms
○ Medication	○ Anxiety	○ Hunger	○ Period
○ Food	○ Reading	○ Insomnia	○ Traveling
○ Weather	○ Noise	○ Smell	○
○ Allergies	○ Motion	○ Sickness	○

RELIEF MEASURES

Medication	
Water	
Sleep	
Exercise	
Other	

Notes

_____

_____

_____

Breakfast

_____
_____
_____
_____

Lunch

_____
_____
_____
_____

Dinner

_____
_____
_____
_____

Snacks/Drinks

_____
_____
_____
_____

Activities

Daily routine: Did you exercise, sleep, travel, etc.

_____
_____
_____
_____
_____
_____
_____
_____
_____
_____
_____

Notes

_____
_____
_____

DATE ____ / ____ / ____	DAY	Mon	Tue	Wed	Thu	Fri	Sat	Sun

Time

Begin		End		Duration	
Begin		End		Duration	
Begin		End		Duration	

Location

☐ Tension ☐ Neck ☐ Migraine ☐ Cluster ☐ Sinus ☐ GCA

Severity

MILD ① ② ③ ④ ⑤ ⑥ ⑦ ⑧ ⑨ ⑩ SEVERE

Triggers

◯ Coffee	◯ Bright light	◯ Eye strain	◯ Commute
◯ Alcohol	◯ Stress	◯ Pc/Tv screen	◯ Pms
◯ Medication	◯ Anxiety	◯ Hunger	◯ Period
◯ Food	◯ Reading	◯ Insomnia	◯ Traveling
◯ Weather	◯ Noise	◯ Smell	◯
◯ Allergies	◯ Motion	◯ Sickness	◯

RELIEF MEASURES

Medication	
Water	
Sleep	
Exercise	
Other	

Notes

_____
_____
_____
_____

Breakfast

_____
_____
_____
_____

Lunch

_____
_____
_____
_____

Dinner

_____
_____
_____
_____

Snacks/Drinks

_____
_____
_____
_____

Activities

Daily routine: Did you exercise, sleep, travel, etc.

_____
_____
_____
_____
_____
_____
_____
_____
_____
_____
_____
_____

Notes

_____
_____
_____

DATE ___/___/___	DAY	Mon	Tue	Wed	Thu	Fri	Sat	Sun

Time

Begin		End		Duration	
Begin		End		Duration	
Begin		End		Duration	

Location

☐ Tension ☐ Neck ☐ Migraine ☐ Cluster ☐ Sinus ☐ GCA

Severity

MILD ① ② ③ ④ ⑤ ⑥ ⑦ ⑧ ⑨ ⑩ SEVERE

Triggers

○ Coffee	○ Bright light	○ Eye strain	○ Commute
○ Alcohol	○ Stress	○ Pc/Tv screen	○ Pms
○ Medication	○ Anxiety	○ Hunger	○ Period
○ Food	○ Reading	○ Insomnia	○ Traveling
○ Weather	○ Noise	○ Smell	○
○ Allergies	○ Motion	○ Sickness	○

RELIEF MEASURES

Medication	
Water	
Sleep	
Exercise	
Other	

Notes

_____
_____
_____
_____

Breakfast

Lunch

Dinner

Snacks/Drinks

Daily routine: Did you exercise, sleep, travel, etc.

DATE ___/___/___	DAY	Mon	Tue	Wed	Thu	Fri	Sat	Sun

Begin		End		Duration	
Begin		End		Duration	
Begin		End		Duration	

Location

☐ Tension ☐ Neck ☐ Migraine ☐ Cluster ☐ Sinus ☐ GCA

Severity

MILD ①②③④⑤⑥⑦⑧⑨⑩ SEVERE

Triggers

○ Coffee	○ Bright light	○ Eye strain	○ Commute
○ Alcohol	○ Stress	○ Pc/Tv screen	○ Pms
○ Medication	○ Anxiety	○ Hunger	○ Period
○ Food	○ Reading	○ Insomnia	○ Traveling
○ Weather	○ Noise	○ Smell	○
○ Allergies	○ Motion	○ Sickness	○

RELIEF MEASURES

Medication	
Water	
Sleep	
Exercise	
Other	

Notes

_____

_____

_____

Breakfast

_____

_____

_____

Lunch

_____

_____

_____

Dinner

_____

_____

_____

Snacks/Drinks

_____

_____

_____

_____

Activities

Daily routine: Did you exercise, sleep, travel, etc.

_____

_____

_____

_____

_____

_____

_____

_____

_____

_____

_____

Notes

_____

_____

_____

DATE ___/___/___	DAY	Mon	Tue	Wed	Thu	Fri	Sat	Sun

Time

Begin		End		Duration	
Begin		End		Duration	
Begin		End		Duration	

Location

☐ Tension ☐ Neck ☐ Migraine ☐ Cluster ☐ Sinus ☐ GCA

Severity

MILD ① ② ③ ④ ⑤ ⑥ ⑦ ⑧ ⑨ ⑩ SEVERE

Triggers

○ Coffee	○ Bright light	○ Eye strain	○ Commute
○ Alcohol	○ Stress	○ Pc/Tv screen	○ Pms
○ Medication	○ Anxiety	○ Hunger	○ Period
○ Food	○ Reading	○ Insomnia	○ Traveling
○ Weather	○ Noise	○ Smell	○
○ Allergies	○ Motion	○ Sickness	○

RELIEF MEASURES

Medication	
Water	
Sleep	
Exercise	
Other	

Notes

_____
_____
_____
_____

Breakfast

Lunch

Dinner

Snacks/Drinks

Daily routine: Did you exercise, sleep, travel, etc.

DATE	___ / ___ / ___	DAY	Mon	Tue	Wed	Thu	Fri	Sat	Sun

Time

Begin		End		Duration	
Begin		End		Duration	
Begin		End		Duration	

Location

☐ Tension ☐ Neck ☐ Migraine ☐ Cluster ☐ Sinus ☐ GCA

Severity

MILD ① ② ③ ④ ⑤ ⑥ ⑦ ⑧ ⑨ ⑩ SEVERE

Triggers

○ Coffee	○ Bright light	○ Eye strain	○ Commute
○ Alcohol	○ Stress	○ Pc/Tv screen	○ Pms
○ Medication	○ Anxiety	○ Hunger	○ Period
○ Food	○ Reading	○ Insomnia	○ Traveling
○ Weather	○ Noise	○ Smell	○
○ Allergies	○ Motion	○ Sickness	○

RELIEF MEASURES

Medication	
Water	
Sleep	
Exercise	
Other	

Notes

_____
_____
_____
_____

Breakfast

Lunch

Dinner

Snacks/Drinks

Daily routine: Did you exercise, sleep, travel, etc.

DATE	/ /	DAY	Mon	Tue	Wed	Thu	Fri	Sat	Sun

Time

Begin		End		Duration	
Begin		End		Duration	
Begin		End		Duration	

Location

☐ Tension ☐ Neck ☐ Migraine ☐ Cluster ☐ Sinus ☐ GCA

Severity

MILD ① ② ③ ④ ⑤ ⑥ ⑦ ⑧ ⑨ ⑩ SEVERE

Triggers

○ Coffee	○ Bright light	○ Eye strain	○ Commute
○ Alcohol	○ Stress	○ Pc/Tv screen	○ Pms
○ Medication	○ Anxiety	○ Hunger	○ Period
○ Food	○ Reading	○ Insomnia	○ Traveling
○ Weather	○ Noise	○ Smell	○
○ Allergies	○ Motion	○ Sickness	○

RELIEF MEASURES

Medication	
Water	
Sleep	
Exercise	
Other	

Notes

_____
_____
_____

Breakfast

Lunch

Dinner

Snacks/Drinks

Daily routine: Did you exercise, sleep, travel, etc.

DATE	___/___/___	DAY	Mon	Tue	Wed	Thu	Fri	Sat	Sun

Time

Begin		End		Duration	
Begin		End		Duration	
Begin		End		Duration	

Location

☐ Tension   ☐ Neck   ☐ Migraine   ☐ Cluster   ☐ Sinus   ☐ GCA

Severity

MILD ① ② ③ ④ ⑤ ⑥ ⑦ ⑧ ⑨ ⑩ SEVERE

Triggers

○ Coffee	○ Bright light	○ Eye strain	○ Commute
○ Alcohol	○ Stress	○ Pc/Tv screen	○ Pms
○ Medication	○ Anxiety	○ Hunger	○ Period
○ Food	○ Reading	○ Insomnia	○ Traveling
○ Weather	○ Noise	○ Smell	○
○ Allergies	○ Motion	○ Sickness	○

RELIEF MEASURES

Medication	
Water	
Sleep	
Exercise	
Other	

Notes

_____
_____
_____

86

Breakfast

_____
_____
_____
_____

Lunch

_____
_____
_____
_____

Dinner

_____
_____
_____
_____

Snacks/Drinks

_____
_____
_____
_____

Activities

Daily routine: Did you exercise, sleep, travel, etc.

_____
_____
_____
_____
_____
_____
_____
_____
_____
_____
_____

Notes

_____
_____
_____

DATE	___/___/___	DAY	Mon	Tue	Wed	Thu	Fri	Sat	Sun

Time

Begin		End		Duration	
Begin		End		Duration	
Begin		End		Duration	

Location

☐ Tension ☐ Neck ☐ Migraine ☐ Cluster ☐ Sinus ☐ GCA

Severity

MILD ① ② ③ ④ ⑤ ⑥ ⑦ ⑧ ⑨ ⑩ SEVERE

Triggers

○ Coffee	○ Bright light	○ Eye strain	○ Commute
○ Alcohol	○ Stress	○ Pc/Tv screen	○ Pms
○ Medication	○ Anxiety	○ Hunger	○ Period
○ Food	○ Reading	○ Insomnia	○ Traveling
○ Weather	○ Noise	○ Smell	○
○ Allergies	○ Motion	○ Sickness	○

RELIEF MEASURES

Medication	
Water	
Sleep	
Exercise	
Other	

Notes

_____
_____
_____

Breakfast

_____
_____
_____
_____

Lunch

_____
_____
_____
_____

Dinner

_____
_____
_____
_____

Snacks/Drinks

_____
_____
_____
_____

Activities

Daily routine: Did you exercise, sleep, travel, etc.

_____
_____
_____
_____
_____
_____
_____
_____
_____
_____

Notes

_____
_____
_____

DATE ___/___/___	DAY	Mon	Tue	Wed	Thu	Fri	Sat	Sun

Time

Begin		End		Duration	
Begin		End		Duration	
Begin		End		Duration	

Location

☐ Tension ☐ Neck ☐ Migraine ☐ Cluster ☐ Sinus ☐ GCA

Severity

MILD ① ② ③ ④ ⑤ ⑥ ⑦ ⑧ ⑨ ⑩ SEVERE

Triggers

○ Coffee	○ Bright light	○ Eye strain	○ Commute
○ Alcohol	○ Stress	○ Pc/Tv screen	○ Pms
○ Medication	○ Anxiety	○ Hunger	○ Period
○ Food	○ Reading	○ Insomnia	○ Traveling
○ Weather	○ Noise	○ Smell	○
○ Allergies	○ Motion	○ Sickness	○

RELIEF MEASURES

Medication	
Water	
Sleep	
Exercise	
Other	

Notes

_____
_____
_____
_____

Breakfast

_____
_____
_____
_____

Lunch

_____
_____
_____
_____

Dinner

_____
_____
_____
_____

Snacks/Drinks

_____
_____
_____
_____

Activities

Daily routine: Did you exercise, sleep, travel, etc.

_____
_____
_____
_____
_____
_____
_____
_____
_____
_____
_____

Notes

_____
_____
_____

DATE	___/___/___	DAY	Mon	Tue	Wed	Thu	Fri	Sat	Sun

Time

Begin		End		Duration	
Begin		End		Duration	
Begin		End		Duration	

Location

☐ Tension ☐ Neck ☐ Migraine ☐ Cluster ☐ Sinus ☐ GCA

Severity

MILD ① ② ③ ④ ⑤ ⑥ ⑦ ⑧ ⑨ ⑩ SEVERE

Triggers

○ Coffee	○ Bright light	○ Eye strain	○ Commute
○ Alcohol	○ Stress	○ Pc/Tv screen	○ Pms
○ Medication	○ Anxiety	○ Hunger	○ Period
○ Food	○ Reading	○ Insomnia	○ Traveling
○ Weather	○ Noise	○ Smell	○
○ Allergies	○ Motion	○ Sickness	○

RELIEF MEASURES

Medication	
Water	
Sleep	
Exercise	
Other	

Notes

_____
_____
_____

Breakfast

_____
_____
_____
_____

Lunch

_____
_____
_____
_____

Dinner

_____
_____
_____
_____

Snacks/Drinks

_____
_____
_____
_____

Activities

Daily routine: Did you exercise, sleep, travel, etc.

_____
_____
_____
_____
_____
_____
_____
_____
_____
_____
_____
_____

Notes

_____
_____
_____

DATE	/ /	DAY	Mon	Tue	Wed	Thu	Fri	Sat	Sun

Time

Begin		End		Duration	
Begin		End		Duration	
Begin		End		Duration	

Location

☐ Tension ☐ Neck ☐ Migraine ☐ Cluster ☐ Sinus ☐ GCA

Severity

MILD ① ② ③ ④ ⑤ ⑥ ⑦ ⑧ ⑨ ⑩ SEVERE

Triggers

○ Coffee	○ Bright light	○ Eye strain	○ Commute
○ Alcohol	○ Stress	○ Pc/Tv screen	○ Pms
○ Medication	○ Anxiety	○ Hunger	○ Period
○ Food	○ Reading	○ Insomnia	○ Traveling
○ Weather	○ Noise	○ Smell	○
○ Allergies	○ Motion	○ Sickness	○

RELIEF MEASURES

Medication	
Water	
Sleep	
Exercise	
Other	

Notes

_____
_____
_____

Breakfast

Lunch

Dinner

Snacks/Drinks

Daily routine: Did you exercise, sleep, travel, etc.

DATE	/ /	DAY	Mon	Tue	Wed	Thu	Fri	Sat	Sun

Time

Begin		End		Duration	
Begin		End		Duration	
Begin		End		Duration	

Location

☐ Tension ☐ Neck ☐ Migraine ☐ Cluster ☐ Sinus ☐ GCA

Severity

MILD ①②③④⑤⑥⑦⑧⑨⑩ SEVERE

Triggers

○ Coffee	○ Bright light	○ Eye strain	○ Commute
○ Alcohol	○ Stress	○ Pc/Tv screen	○ Pms
○ Medication	○ Anxiety	○ Hunger	○ Period
○ Food	○ Reading	○ Insomnia	○ Traveling
○ Weather	○ Noise	○ Smell	○
○ Allergies	○ Motion	○ Sickness	○

RELIEF MEASURES

Medication	
Water	
Sleep	
Exercise	
Other	

Notes

_____
_____
_____

Breakfast

Lunch

Dinner

Snacks/Drinks

Daily routine: Did you exercise, sleep, travel, etc.

DATE ___ / ___ / ___	DAY	Mon	Tue	Wed	Thu	Fri	Sat	Sun

Begin		End		Duration	
Begin		End		Duration	
Begin		End		Duration	

Location

☐ Tension ☐ Neck ☐ Migraine ☐ Cluster ☐ Sinus ☐ GCA

Severity

MILD ① ② ③ ④ ⑤ ⑥ ⑦ ⑧ ⑨ ⑩ SEVERE

Triggers

○ Coffee	○ Bright light	○ Eye strain	○ Commute
○ Alcohol	○ Stress	○ Pc/Tv screen	○ Pms
○ Medication	○ Anxiety	○ Hunger	○ Period
○ Food	○ Reading	○ Insomnia	○ Traveling
○ Weather	○ Noise	○ Smell	○
○ Allergies	○ Motion	○ Sickness	○

RELIEF MEASURES

Medication	
Water	
Sleep	
Exercise	
Other	

Notes

_____
_____
_____
_____

Breakfast

_____
_____
_____
_____

Lunch

_____
_____
_____
_____

Dinner

_____
_____
_____
_____

Snacks/Drinks

_____
_____
_____
_____

Activities

Daily routine: Did you exercise, sleep, travel, etc.

_____
_____
_____
_____
_____
_____
_____
_____
_____
_____
_____
_____

Notes

_____
_____
_____

DATE	___/___/___	DAY	Mon	Tue	Wed	Thu	Fri	Sat	Sun

Time

Begin		End		Duration	
Begin		End		Duration	
Begin		End		Duration	

Location

☐ Tension ☐ Neck ☐ Migraine ☐ Cluster ☐ Sinus ☐ GCA

Severity

MILD ① ② ③ ④ ⑤ ⑥ ⑦ ⑧ ⑨ ⑩ SEVERE

Triggers

◯ Coffee	◯ Bright light	◯ Eye strain	◯ Commute
◯ Alcohol	◯ Stress	◯ Pc/Tv screen	◯ Pms
◯ Medication	◯ Anxiety	◯ Hunger	◯ Period
◯ Food	◯ Reading	◯ Insomnia	◯ Traveling
◯ Weather	◯ Noise	◯ Smell	◯
◯ Allergies	◯ Motion	◯ Sickness	◯

RELIEF MEASURES

Medication	
Water	
Sleep	
Exercise	
Other	

Notes

_____
_____
_____
_____

Breakfast

Lunch

Dinner

Snacks/Drinks

Daily routine: Did you exercise, sleep, travel, etc.

DATE	___/___/___	DAY	Mon	Tue	Wed	Thu	Fri	Sat	Sun

Time

Begin		End		Duration	
Begin		End		Duration	
Begin		End		Duration	

Location

☐ Tension ☐ Neck ☐ Migraine ☐ Cluster ☐ Sinus ☐ GCA

Severity

MILD ① ② ③ ④ ⑤ ⑥ ⑦ ⑧ ⑨ ⑩ SEVERE

Triggers

◯ Coffee	◯ Bright light	◯ Eye strain	◯ Commute
◯ Alcohol	◯ Stress	◯ Pc/Tv screen	◯ Pms
◯ Medication	◯ Anxiety	◯ Hunger	◯ Period
◯ Food	◯ Reading	◯ Insomnia	◯ Traveling
◯ Weather	◯ Noise	◯ Smell	◯
◯ Allergies	◯ Motion	◯ Sickness	◯

RELIEF MEASURES

Medication	
Water	
Sleep	
Exercise	
Other	

Notes

_____
_____
_____
_____

Breakfast

_____

_____

_____

Lunch

_____

_____

_____

Dinner

_____

_____

_____

Snacks/Drinks

_____

_____

_____

_____

Activities

Daily routine: Did you exercise, sleep, travel, etc.

_____

_____

_____

_____

_____

_____

_____

_____

_____

_____

_____

Notes

_____

_____

_____

_____

DATE ___/___/___	DAY	Mon	Tue	Wed	Thu	Fri	Sat	Sun

Time

Begin		End		Duration	
Begin		End		Duration	
Begin		End		Duration	

Location

☐ Tension   ☐ Neck   ☐ Migraine   ☐ Cluster   ☐ Sinus   ☐ GCA

Severity

MILD ① ② ③ ④ ⑤ ⑥ ⑦ ⑧ ⑨ ⑩ SEVERE

Triggers

○ Coffee	○ Bright light	○ Eye strain	○ Commute
○ Alcohol	○ Stress	○ Pc/Tv screen	○ Pms
○ Medication	○ Anxiety	○ Hunger	○ Period
○ Food	○ Reading	○ Insomnia	○ Traveling
○ Weather	○ Noise	○ Smell	○
○ Allergies	○ Motion	○ Sickness	○

RELIEF MEASURES

Medication	
Water	
Sleep	
Exercise	
Other	

Notes

_____
_____
_____
_____

104

Breakfast

Lunch

Dinner

Snacks/Drinks

Daily routine: Did you exercise, sleep, travel, etc.

DATE	___/___/___	DAY	Mon	Tue	Wed	Thu	Fri	Sat	Sun

Time

Begin		End		Duration	
Begin		End		Duration	
Begin		End		Duration	

Location

☐ Tension ☐ Neck ☐ Migraine ☐ Cluster ☐ Sinus ☐ GCA

Severity

MILD ①②③④⑤⑥⑦⑧⑨⑩ SEVERE

Triggers

○ Coffee	○ Bright light	○ Eye strain	○ Commute
○ Alcohol	○ Stress	○ Pc/Tv screen	○ Pms
○ Medication	○ Anxiety	○ Hunger	○ Period
○ Food	○ Reading	○ Insomnia	○ Traveling
○ Weather	○ Noise	○ Smell	○
○ Allergies	○ Motion	○ Sickness	○

RELIEF MEASURES

Medication	
Water	
Sleep	
Exercise	
Other	

Notes

_____
_____
_____
_____

Breakfast

_____
_____
_____
_____

Lunch

_____
_____
_____
_____

Dinner

_____
_____
_____
_____

Snacks/Drinks

_____
_____
_____
_____

Activities

Daily routine: Did you exercise, sleep, travel, etc.

_____
_____
_____
_____
_____
_____
_____
_____
_____
_____
_____

Notes

_____
_____
_____

Made in the USA
Monee, IL
18 April 2022

94990329R00059